PLANT BASED COOKBOOK FOR WOMEN

Easy, Nutritious, and Delicious Plant-Based Recipes for a Healthy Lifestyle

Teresa Gilmore

TABLE OF CONTENT

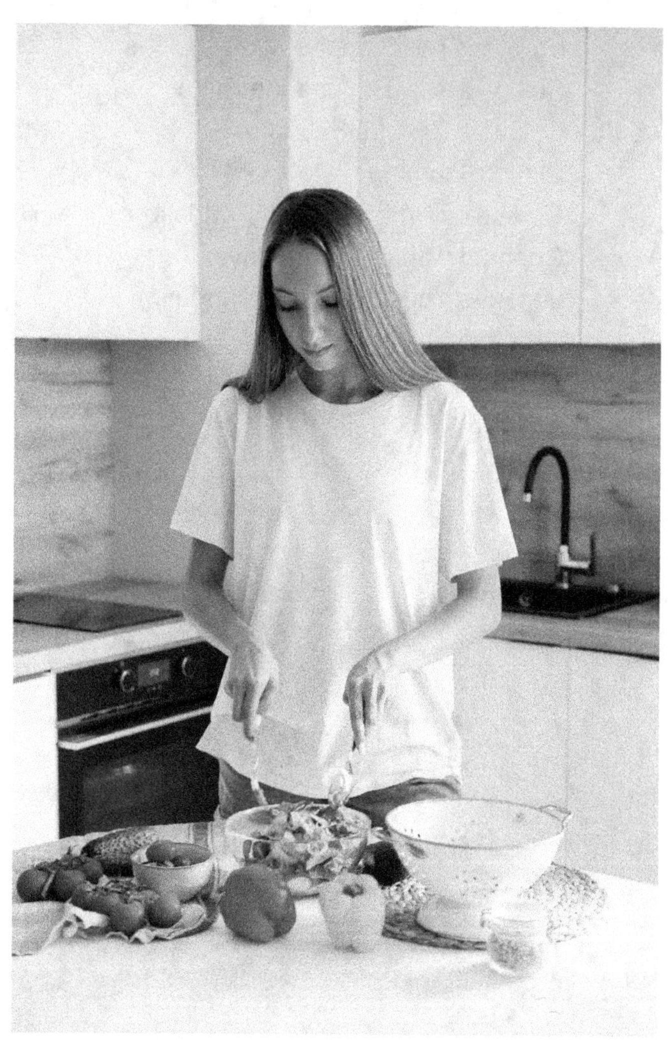

INTRODUCTION

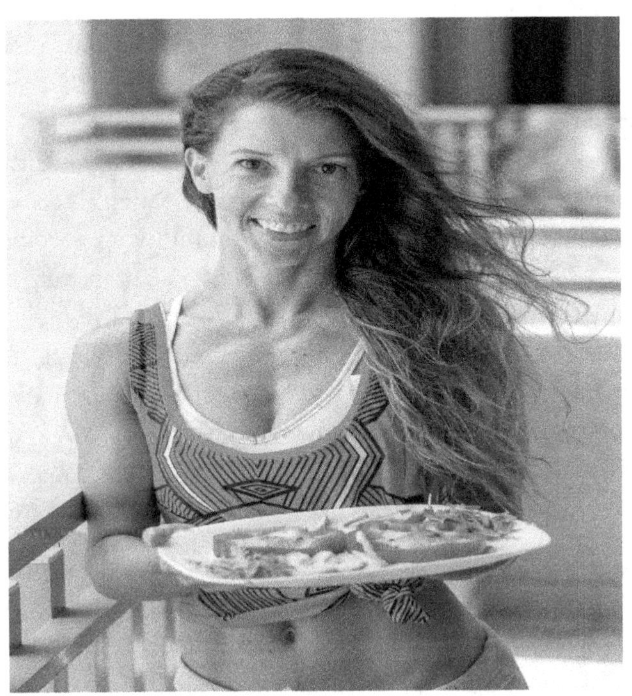

Embracing "Harmony on the Plate"

In a world marked by the constant hustle and bustle, women often find themselves at the epicenter of myriad responsibilities—balancing careers, family, and personal pursuits. In this dynamic landscape, the essence of self-care can easily be overshadowed, and the importance of nurturing one's well-being can be inadvertently neglected. It is within this context that "Harmony on the Plate: A Plant-Based Cookbook for Women" emerges as a beacon, inviting women to reclaim a fundamental aspect of their lives—their relationship with food.

The concept of harmony goes beyond the mere amalgamation of ingredients; it extends into the very essence of well-being. This cookbook is not just a collection of recipes; it's a guide to cultivating balance, simplicity, and joy through plant-based eating. It serves as a testament to the idea that healthful living need not be complex or time-consuming, but rather, it can be woven seamlessly into the fabric of everyday life.

The decision to embrace a plant-based lifestyle is not merely a culinary choice; it is a commitment to vitality, compassion, and environmental stewardship. As we embark on this culinary journey together, the pages of "Harmony on the Plate" unfold to reveal a thoughtful exploration of the benefits that plant-based eating specifically holds for women.

The Healthful Benefits for Women

Women's health is a nuanced tapestry, influenced by physiological intricacies that demand unique nutritional considerations. "Harmony on the Plate" delves into the wealth of benefits that plant-based eating offers in promoting women's well-being.

Plant-based diets are inherently rich in essential nutrients, providing a broad spectrum of vitamins, minerals, and antioxidants crucial for women's health. From supporting bone density with plant-based calcium sources to fostering hormonal balance through phytoestrogens, each recipe in this cookbook is designed with a keen understanding of the nutritional needs that accompany different stages of a woman's life.

Beyond the physical realm, the mental and emotional dimensions of well-being are integral components addressed within these pages. Plant-based eating has been associated with improved mood, increased energy levels, and enhanced mental clarity. Recognizing the interconnectedness of mind and body, "Harmony on the Plate" emphasizes the role of wholesome, plant-based nutrition in cultivating a holistic sense of wellness for women.

A Culinary Journey to Simplicity

In the midst of busy schedules and demanding routines, the notion of preparing healthful meals can often feel like an insurmountable challenge. Here, the cookbook becomes a culinary ally, introducing a harmonious fusion of simplicity and nutritional richness. Each recipe is crafted with the understanding that time is a precious commodity, and yet, the desire for nourishing, delicious meals remains unwavering.

The simplicity embedded in these recipes is not a compromise; it is an intentional choice to make healthful eating accessible to women from all walks of life. From the vibrant salads that come together with minimal effort to the one-pot wonders that simplify dinnertime, "Harmony on the Plate" redefines the notion that nutritious cooking must be arduous.

Inviting Women Back to the Kitchen:

"Harmony on the Plate" extends an invitation to women to rediscover the joy of the kitchen—a space often overlooked in the relentless pursuit of daily obligations. This cookbook is a celebration of the kitchen as a sanctuary, a place where the act of preparing meals becomes a nourishing ritual and a form of self-care.

In this introduction, we embark on a journey that transcends the boundaries of conventional cookbooks. "Harmony on the Plate" is not just about what's on the plate; it's about the experience of creating, savoring, and embracing a lifestyle that harmonizes health, simplicity, and pleasure. As we turn the pages, may each recipe be a step towards a more vibrant, balanced, and joyful life for women—because true harmony begins on the plate. No

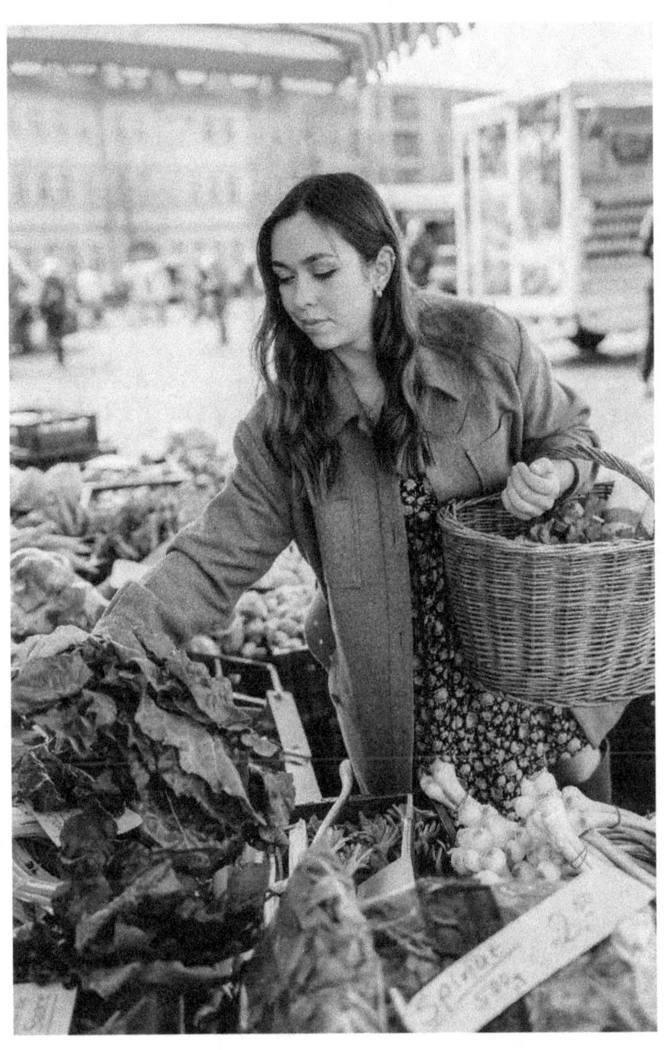

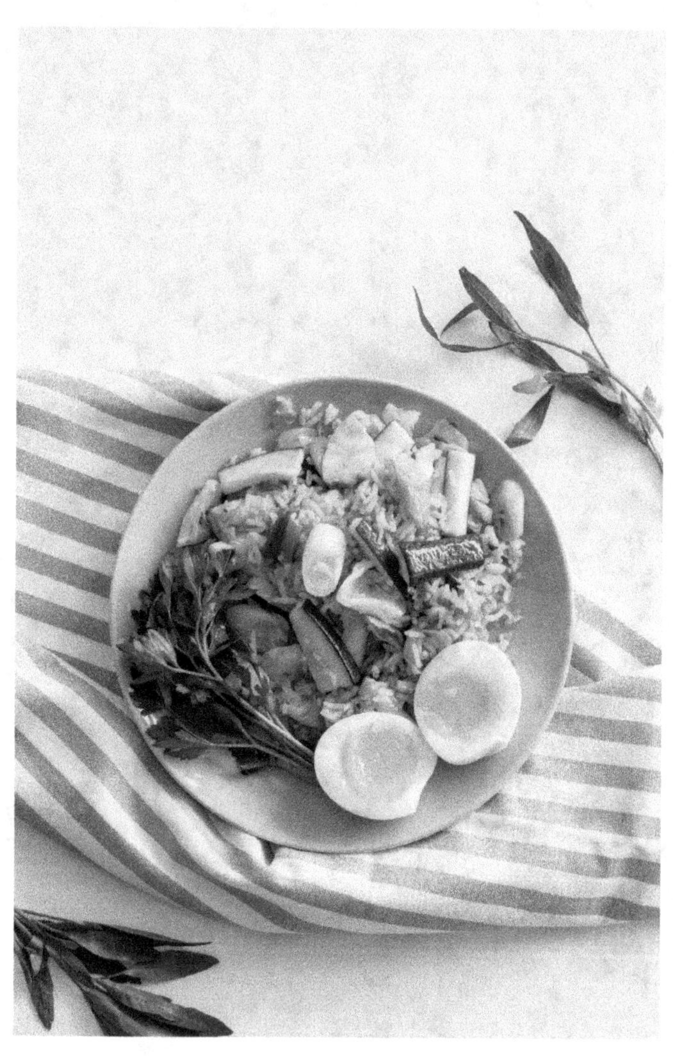

CHAPTER ONE

Getting Started: Cultivating Wellness in Every Bite

Embarking on a plant-based journey is a transformative decision—one that holds the promise of holistic well-being and a vibrant, healthful life. As you stand at the threshold of this culinary adventure with "A Plant-Based Cookbook for Women," the getting started section becomes your compass, guiding you through the essential steps to infuse your daily life with the nourishing power of plant-based eating.

Kitchen Essentials for Plant-Based Cooking:

The heart of any culinary undertaking lies in a well-equipped kitchen. In this section, we unravel the fundamental tools and ingredients that will be your allies on this plant-based voyage. From versatile kitchen gadgets that streamline meal preparation to pantry staples that form the backbone of healthful recipes, you'll discover that creating a plant-based kitchen need not be an overwhelming task. Instead, it's an empowering step toward crafting meals that are as practical as they are delicious.

Consider the knife as your artist's brush, transforming vibrant vegetables into culinary masterpieces. Embrace the cutting board as your canvas, and let the colors of nature inspire your creations. The blender becomes a symphony conductor, blending flavors and textures into harmonious delights. As you delve into this section, you'll not only equip your kitchen but also awaken the artist within, ready to paint your plate with the hues of health and vitality.

Stocking a Balanced Pantry:

A plant-based pantry is the cornerstone of successful and sustainable plant-based living. It's not merely about replacing animal products with plant alternatives; it's about curating a pantry that supports your well-being while unleashing a world of flavors. From whole grains and legumes to an array of spices and herbs, each ingredient plays a crucial role in crafting nutritionally rich and delicious meals.

"Harmony on the Plate" guides you through the art of stocking a balanced pantry—one that reflects your commitment to health and aligns with the versatility of plant-based cooking. Discover the nutritional powerhouse of quinoa, the protein-packed elegance of lentils, and the wholesome goodness of ancient grains. Unearth the magic of herbs and spices that elevate your dishes, turning every meal into a sensory experience.

As you open your pantry to a world of plant-based possibilities, you'll find that the journey of healthful living is not about deprivation but abundance. It's about exploring the diverse flavors and textures that plant-based ingredients bring to the table, creating a tapestry of culinary delight that resonates with both your taste buds and your well-being.

Empowering Your Culinary Journey

Getting started with a plant-based lifestyle is more than a practical consideration—it's a mindset shift. It's about viewing the kitchen not as a place of routine, but as a canvas for creativity and self-care. It's an invitation to explore, experiment, and savor the transformative power of each ingredient.

This section is a testament to empowerment, reminding you that every choice you make in your kitchen is a step toward a more vibrant and healthful existence. Whether you're a seasoned chef or taking your first steps into the world of plant-based cooking, "Harmony on the Plate" empowers you to take control of your well-being, one delicious and nutritious bite at a time.

As you absorb the wisdom and practical insights within the getting started section, let it be a prelude to the symphony of health, joy, and fulfillment that awaits you in the pages of this plant-based cookbook for women. Your journey has begun, and each step is a celebration of the remarkable harmony that unfolds when you choose wellness in every bite.

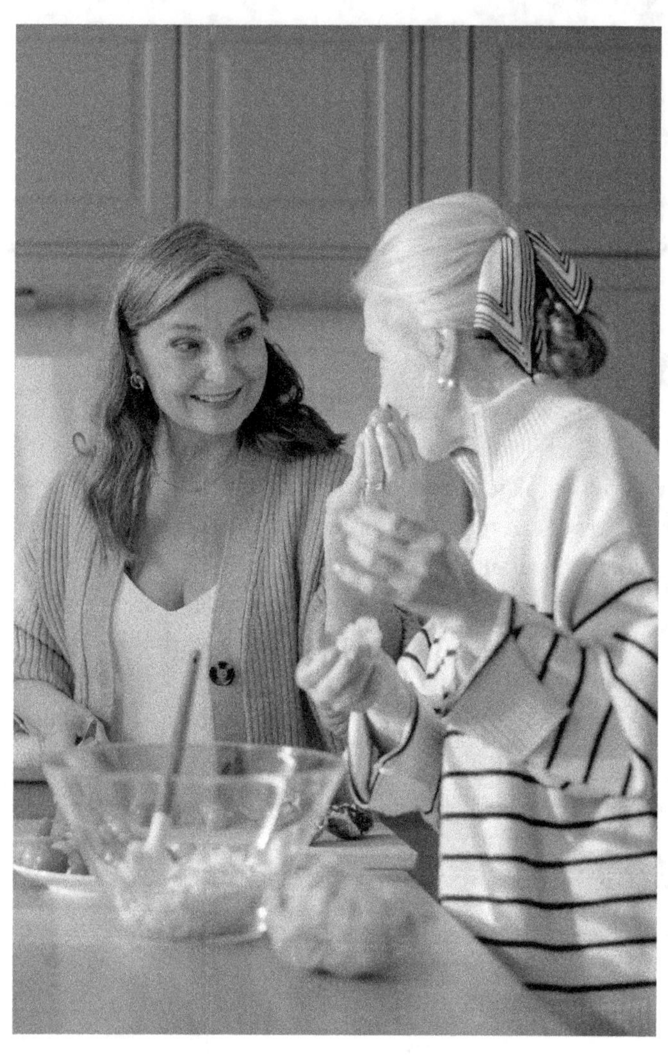

CHAPTER TWO

Breakfast Delights: Elevating Women's Wellness One Bite at a Time

In the mosaic of a woman's day, breakfast stands as a powerful canvas—a moment to cultivate energy, nourishment, and a vibrant start to the day. "Harmony on the Plate: A Plant-Based Cookbook for Women" curates a symphony of Breakfast Delights, where each recipe is not just a meal but a celebration of health, joy, and the holistic well-being of women.

1. Energizing Smoothie Bowls: Bursting with Color and Vitality

Dive into the world of Energizing Smoothie Bowls, where each spoonful is a journey into the heart of healthful living. The Berry Bliss Bowl combines the antioxidant prowess of mixed berries with the creamy goodness of almond butter, creating a burst of flavor that awakens your taste buds. For a tropical escape, the Mango Tango Bowl invites the vibrancy of mango, pineapple, and coconut into a dance of flavors, transporting you to a paradise of wellness. These bowls not only tantalize the taste buds but also infuse your morning with a spectrum of nutrients, setting the stage for a day of vitality.

2. Wholesome Overnight Oats: A Symphony of Simplicity and Sustenance

In the rush of morning routines, Wholesome Overnight Oats emerge as a time-saving marvel that doesn't compromise on nutrition or taste. The Classic Berry Bliss Oats weave together oats, almond milk, and a medley of fresh berries, creating a delightful harmony of chewiness and juiciness. For a cozy twist, the Cinnamon Apple Pie Oats embrace the comforting warmth of apples and spices, making your breakfast a comforting hug in a bowl. These overnight oats recipes not only simplify your mornings but also provide a nutrient-packed foundation for the day ahead.

3. Nutrient-Packed Avocado Toast Variations: Elevating the Everyday Staple

Avocado toast, a beloved classic, takes on new dimensions in "Plant based cookbook for women," becoming a canvas for nutrient-packed creativity. The Green Goddess Avocado Toast combines creamy avocado with nutrient-rich greens, creating a powerhouse of vitamins and minerals. For a protein boost, the Smoky Chickpea Avocado Toast introduces a layer of seasoned chickpeas, infusing your breakfast with plant-powered sustenance. These variations not only redefine the art of avocado toast but also cater to the specific nutritional needs of women, ensuring a balanced and delicious start to the day.

4. Superfood Parfait: A Luxurious Indulgence in Wellness

Step into the realm of indulgence with the Superfood Parfait—a breakfast option that marries decadence with nutritional richness. The Berry Chia Parfait layers antioxidant-rich berries with chia seed pudding, creating a visually stunning and nutritionally dense delight. For a touch of exoticism, the Tropical Turmeric Parfait introduces the anti-inflammatory benefits of turmeric amid layers of tropical fruits and coconut yogurt. These parfaits not only pamper your taste buds but also provide a luxurious dose of wellness, turning your breakfast into a daily celebration of self-care.

In this plant based cookbook, each breakfast recipe is crafted with the understanding that women deserve a morning ritual that goes beyond sustenance—it should be a source of joy, empowerment, and holistic well-being. These Breakfast Delights invite you to savor the exquisite symphony of flavors, textures, and nutrients, making each bite a declaration of self-love and a powerful step towards a day filled with energy and vitality.

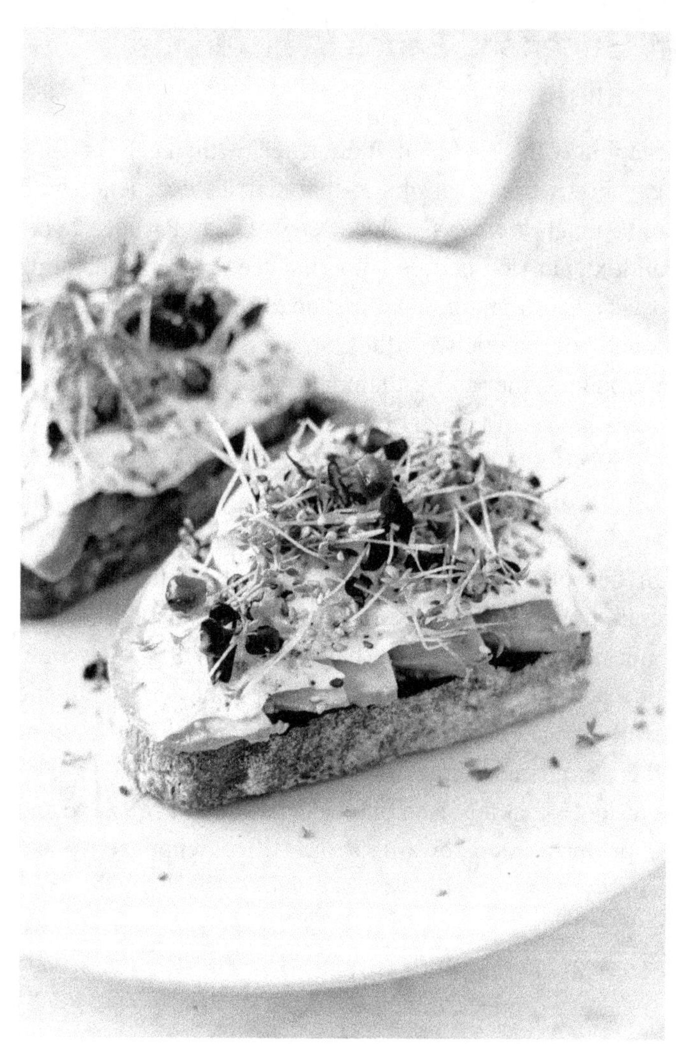

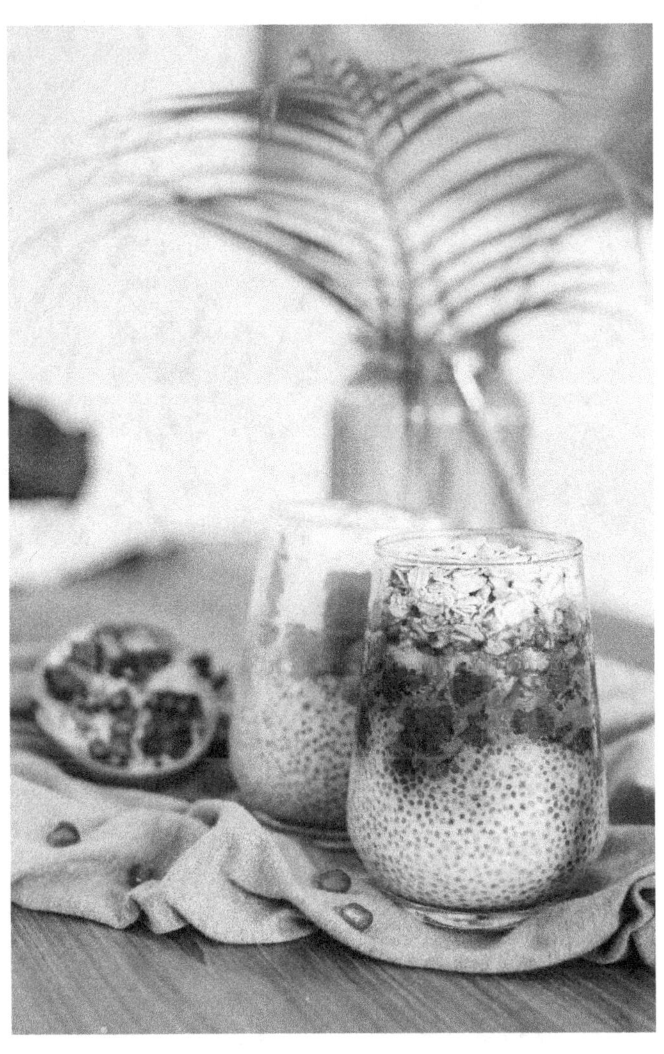

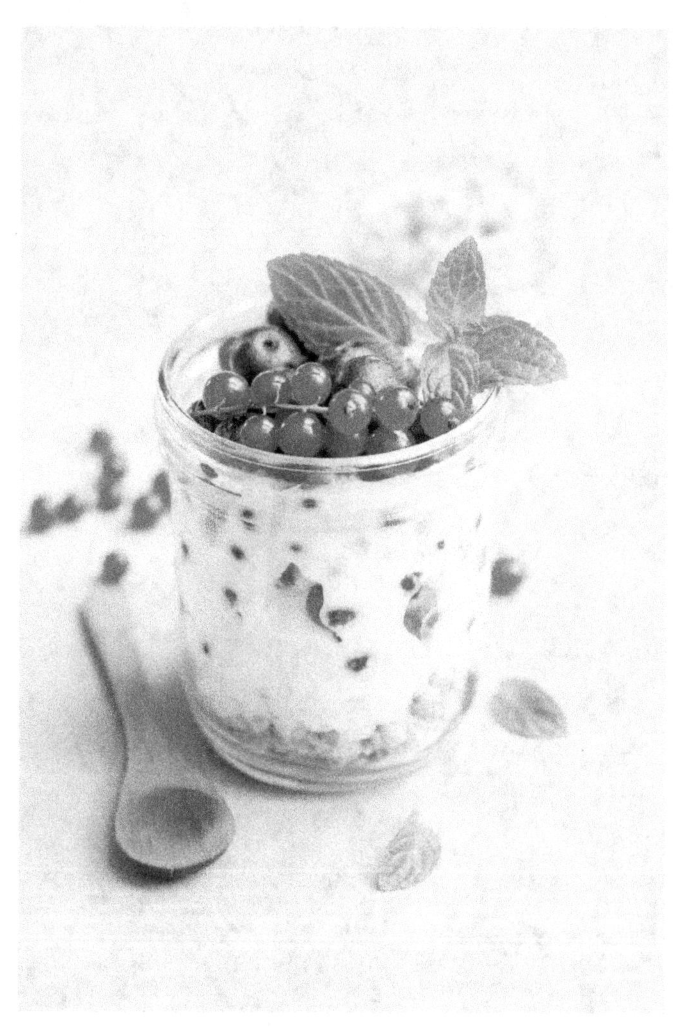

CHAPTER THREE

Lunchtime Nourishment: A Symphony of Healthful Choices for Women

In the cadence of a woman's day, lunchtime stands as a pivotal moment—a respite to refuel, recharge, and savor the nourishment that fuels the afternoon endeavors. "Harmony on the Plate: A Plant-Based Cookbook for Women" orchestrates a harmonious lunchtime experience, where each recipe becomes a melody of flavors, textures, and healthful choices tailored to empower and energize women.

1. Vibrant Salad Creations: A Palette of Wellness on Your Plate

Salads, often underestimated, take center stage in this symphony of lunchtime nourishment. The Garden Goddess Salad is a celebration of crisp greens, nutrient-packed vegetables, and a burst of color from cherry tomatoes and bell peppers. For a protein boost, the Powerhouse Quinoa Salad combines the ancient grain with chickpeas, avocado, and a zesty lemon-tahini dressing. These vibrant salads not only tantalize the taste buds but also deliver a medley of vitamins, minerals, and antioxidants, aligning with women's unique nutritional needs.

2. Hearty Quinoa and Grain Bowls: A Wholesome Harmony of Ingredients

Quinoa and grain bowls emerge as the heartwarming protagonists of a healthful lunch. The Mediterranean Quinoa Bowl introduces a melody of olives, cucumbers, and sun-dried tomatoes, invoking the flavors of the Mediterranean coast. For a taste of the East, the Teriyaki Tempeh Grain Bowl combines nutty quinoa with vibrant vegetables and marinated tempeh. These bowls not only satisfy your taste buds but also provide a satisfying blend of proteins, fibers, and essential nutrients, making your lunch a source of sustained energy and vitality.

3. Quick and Flavorful Wraps: A Symphony of Portable Delights

For women on the go, the Quick and Flavorful Wraps in "Harmony on the Plate" offer a convenient yet healthful lunchtime solution. The Mediterranean Chickpea Wrap layers hummus, crisp vegetables, and chickpea patties in a whole-grain wrap, creating a portable feast of Mediterranean flavors. The Spicy Peanut Tofu Wrap introduces a fusion of Asian-inspired flavors with marinated tofu, crunchy veggies, and a zesty peanut sauce. These wraps not only provide a delectable break from routine but also ensure that your lunchtime is both satisfying and health-conscious.

4. Elegant Plant-Based Entrées: Culinary Artistry for Lunch

Lunchtime becomes an occasion for culinary artistry with the Elegant Plant-Based Entrées in this cookbook. The Stuffed Bell Peppers with Quinoa and Black Beans offer a colorful and flavorful twist to the traditional stuffed peppers, showcasing the versatility of plant-based ingredients. For a taste of Italy, the Eggplant and Tomato Tower combines layers of roasted eggplant and tomato with a savory basil pesto. These entrées not only elevate your lunch to a gourmet experience but also embrace the sophistication of healthful living. This plant based cookbook guides women to relish lunchtime as a moment of self-care and empowerment. These lunchtime nourishment recipes are not merely about filling a hunger gap; they are about crafting a meal that aligns with the unique needs of women. As you savor each bite of these healthful creations, let it be a reminder that lunchtime can be a celebration—an affirmation of your well-being, vitality, and the beauty of choosing a plant-powered path to nourishment.

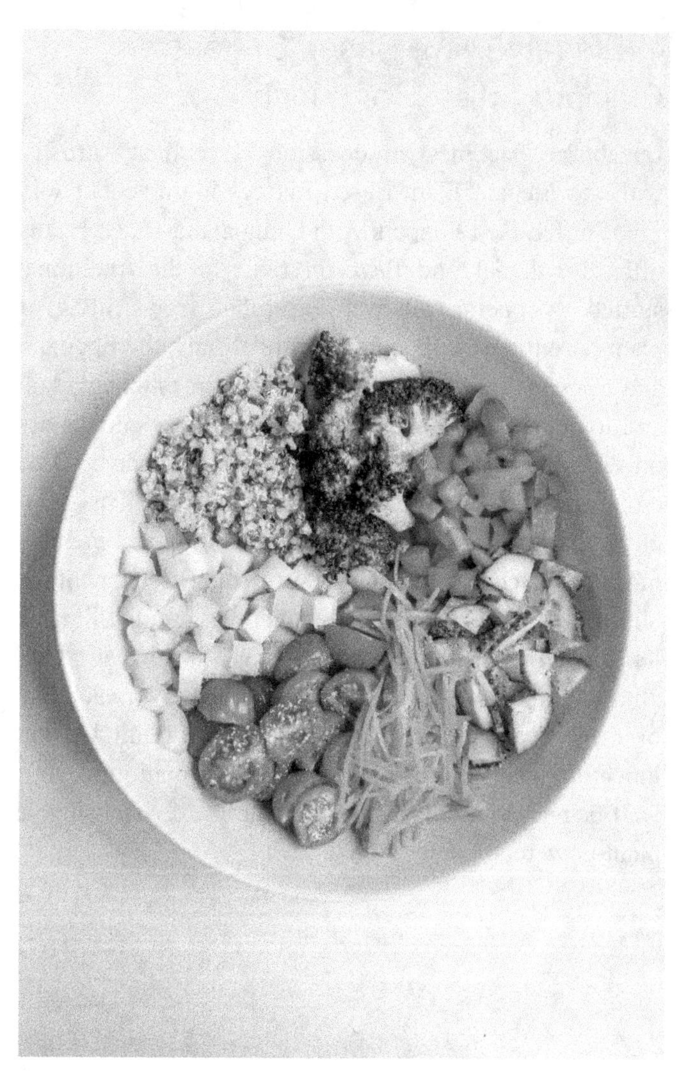

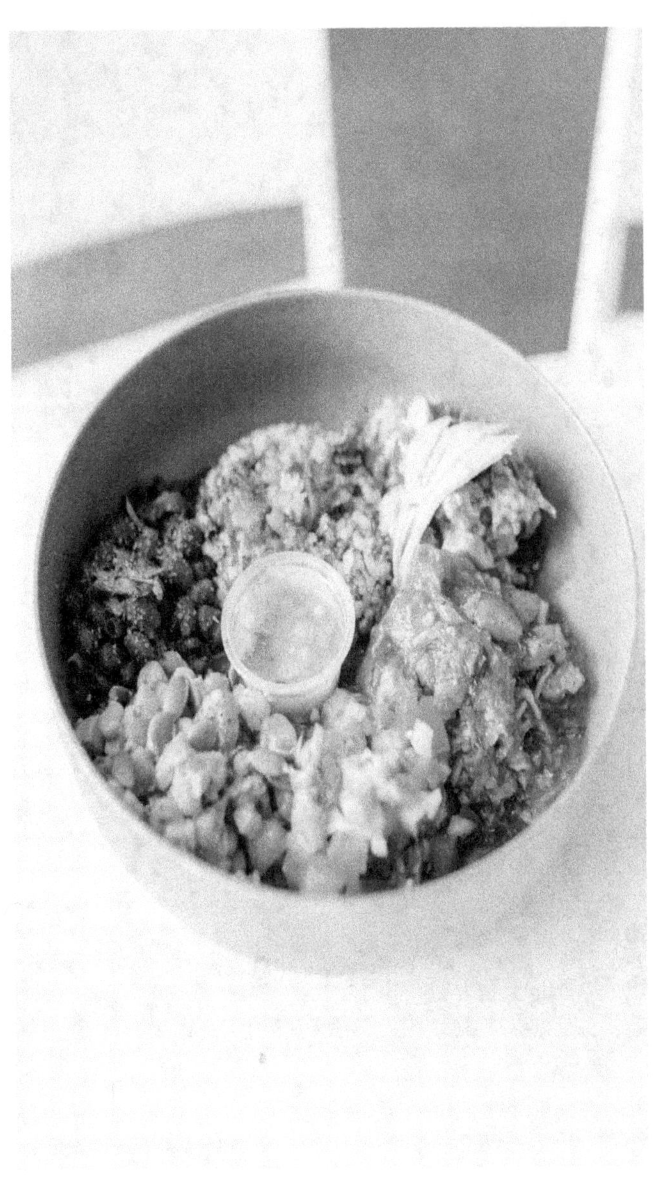

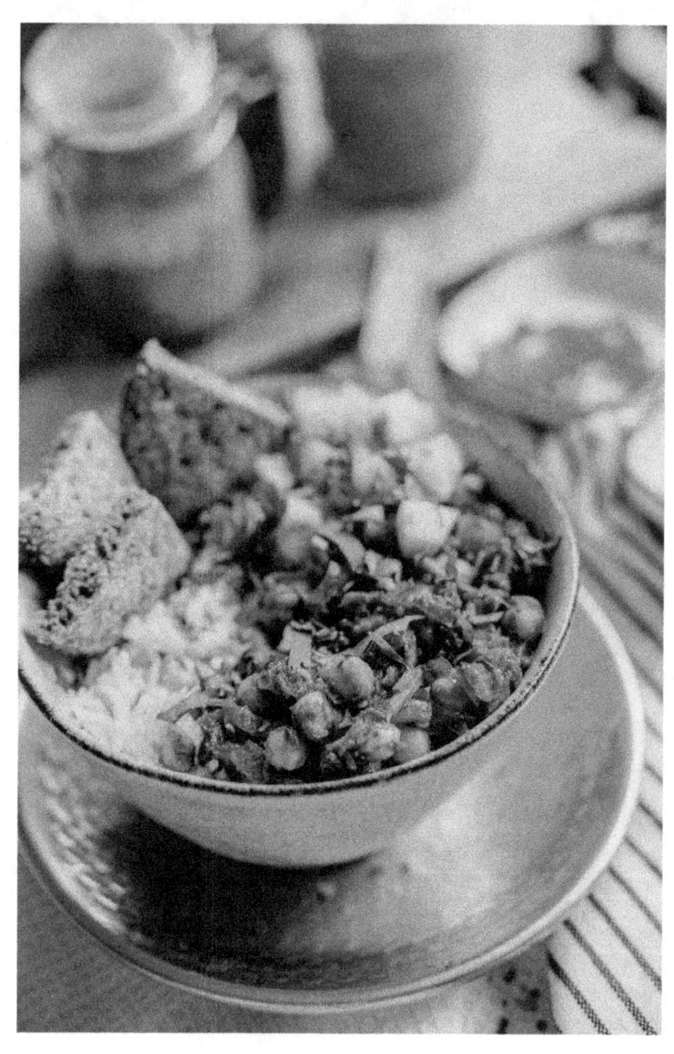

CHAPTER FOUR

Dinnertime Harmony: A Symphony of Healthful Indulgence for Women

As the day gently transitions into evening, dinnertime becomes a sanctuary—a moment to unwind, reflect, and savor the culmination of the day's energy. In "Harmony on the Plate: A Plant-Based Cookbook for Women," the chapter on Dinnertime Harmony unfolds as a captivating symphony of flavors, textures, and healthful choices, crafting an evening experience that nourishes both body and soul.

1. One-Pot Wonders for Busy Evenings: Effortless Elegance on Your Plate

For women navigating the demands of life, One-Pot Wonders offer a culinary solution that blends simplicity with sophistication. The Tuscan White Bean Stew introduces a rustic harmony of cannellini beans, kale, and tomatoes simmered in aromatic herbs and spices. The Coconut Curry Lentil Pot unites red lentils with a medley of vegetables in a rich coconut curry sauce. These one-pot creations not only minimize cleanup but also infuse your evening with comforting aromas and a symphony of nourishing ingredients.

2. Satisfying Stir-Fries and Skillets: Culinary Artistry in Motion

Stir-Fries and Skillets emerge as the dynamic maestros of dinnertime, orchestrating a dance of vibrant colors and bold flavors. The Ginger Sesame Tofu Stir-Fry introduces crispy tofu paired with a rainbow of vegetables, all bathed in a savory ginger sesame sauce. The Quinoa Veggie Skillet combines fluffy quinoa with an array of sautéed vegetables, creating a satisfying melody of textures. These recipes not only bring excitement to your dinner table but also ensure a balanced blend of proteins, fibers, and essential nutrients, aligning with the nutritional needs of women.

3. Elegant Plant-Based Entrées: Elevating Your Evening Feast

Dinnertime transforms into a culinary spectacle with Elegant Plant-Based Entrées that embrace the art of indulgence. The Stuffed Portobello Mushrooms with Spinach and Artichokes offer a sophisticated blend of flavors and textures, creating a savory masterpiece. For a taste of the Mediterranean, the Lemon Herb Baked Zucchini boats showcase the simplicity and elegance of fresh ingredients. These entrées transcend the ordinary, providing women with a dining experience that harmonizes healthful choices with gourmet delight.

4. Wholesome Pasta Creations: Comforting Indulgence with a Healthful Twist

Pasta, a timeless favorite, takes center stage in the Wholesome Pasta Creations of "Harmony on the Plate." The Creamy Avocado and Cherry Tomato Linguine introduces a luscious avocado-based sauce, bringing a creamy texture without the need for dairy. The Spinach and Chickpea Penne highlights the protein-packed goodness of chickpeas amid the comforting embrace of whole-grain pasta. These pasta creations offer a comforting indulgence that does not compromise on nutrition, ensuring that your dinnertime is both satisfying and health-conscious.

5. Flavorful Grain Bowls: A Wholesome Medley in a Bowl

Grain Bowls become a canvas for culinary expression, allowing you to craft a personalized masterpiece with an array of wholesome ingredients. The Mediterranean Quinoa Bowl returns, this time as a dinner option, marrying the flavors of olives, tomatoes, and artichokes with quinoa. The Teriyaki Tempeh Grain Bowl evolves into a heartier rendition for the evening, showcasing the umami goodness of marinated tempeh. These grain bowls not only cater to your taste preferences but also offer a customizable approach to healthful dinnertime indulgence.

As you explore the recipes in the Dinnertime Harmony chapter, let it be a reminder that dinner is not just a meal—it's a celebration of the day's triumphs and an opportunity to honor your well-being. These healthful and indulgent recipes ensure that your evenings are filled with not just nourishment but also the joy of savoring every bite in the harmonious embrace of a plant-powered feast.

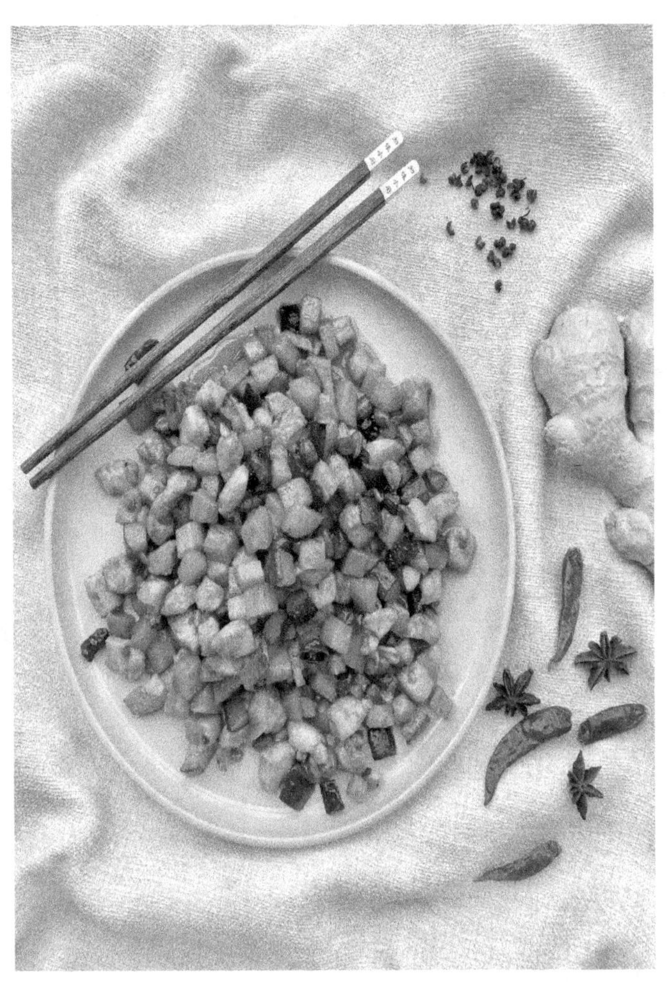

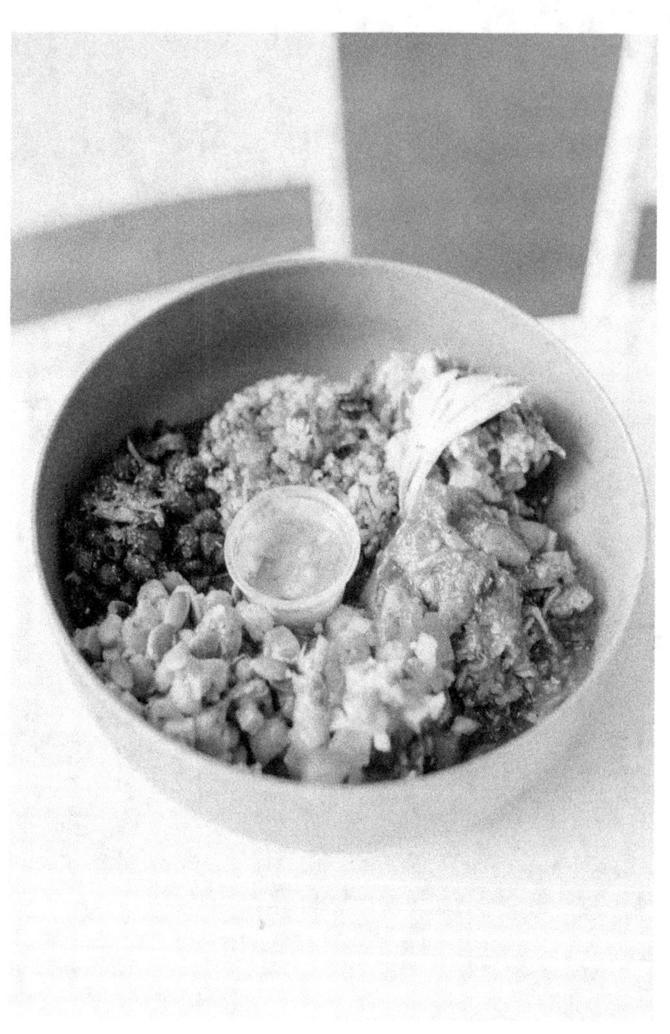

CHAPTER FIVE

Snacks & Appetizers: A Symphony of Wholesome Indulgence for Women

In the melody of a woman's day, snacks and appetizers become the playful interlude—a moment to satiate cravings with flavors that dance on the palate while embracing the commitment to health. The Plant-Based Cookbook for Women unfolds a captivating chapter on Snacks & Appetizers, where each recipe is a note in the symphony of healthful indulgence tailored to empower and energize women.

1. Guilt-Free Guacamole and Salsas: A Fiesta of Fresh Flavors

Enter a realm of vibrant hues and fresh flavors with Guilt-Free Guacamole and Salsas that redefine snacking. The Classic Guacamole weaves together ripe avocados, tomatoes, onions, and a burst of citrus—a creamy dip that nourishes while tantalizing your taste buds. For a spicy kick, the Mango Salsa introduces the sweetness of mangoes harmonized with jalapeños and cilantro. These guilt-free delights not only satisfy your craving for a savory snack but also deliver a host of essential nutrients, making them perfect for women seeking a healthful indulgence.

2. Baked Veggie Chips and Dips: Crispy Delights without the Guilt

Turn snacking into a guilt-free affair with Baked Veggie Chips and Dips that redefine the notion of crunchy delights. The Sweet Potato Chips introduce a colorful array of nutrients with the natural sweetness of sweet potatoes and a touch of savory spices. Pair them with the Creamy Spinach Artichoke Dip for a harmonious blend of flavors and textures that elevate your snacking experience. These baked delights offer a satisfying crunch without compromising on health, ensuring women can savor the joy of snacking with a wholesome twist.

3. Savory Bites for Any Occasion: Small Pleasures, Big Flavors

Savory Bites take center stage in this culinary journey, offering small pleasures that pack a punch of flavor. The Stuffed Mushroom Caps with Herbed Quinoa are elegant morsels filled with protein-rich quinoa, herbs, and a hint of garlic. For a Mediterranean twist, the Olive and Sun-Dried Tomato Tapenade on Crostini invites you to savor the bold flavors of the Mediterranean in every bite. These savory bites not only serve as delightful appetizers but also showcase the artistry of crafting healthful and flavorful snacks.

4. Nutrient-Packed Hummus Variations: A Wholesome Dip into Flavor

Hummus, a beloved classic, takes on new dimensions with Nutrient-Packed Hummus Variations that transform snacking into a delightful ritual. The Roasted Red Pepper Hummus offers a vibrant twist with the smoky sweetness of roasted peppers. For an earthy experience, the Beetroot and Walnut Hummus introduces a burst of color and nutty richness. Pair these hummus variations with vegetable sticks or whole-grain crackers for a snack that satisfies both cravings and nutritional needs, ensuring women can indulge without compromise.

5. Sweet and Savory Energy Balls: Power-Packed Bites for On-the-Go

Elevate your snacking with Sweet and Savory Energy Balls, power-packed bites that energize and satiate. The Almond Date Energy Balls combine the sweetness of dates with the nutty richness of almonds, creating a wholesome treat. For a savory twist, the Mediterranean Olive and Herb Energy Balls showcase the savory flavors of olives and herbs in a convenient, bite-sized form. These energy balls offer a convenient and nutritious solution for on-the-go snacking, empowering women to fuel their busy lives with healthful indulgence. As you explore the recipes in the Snacks & Appetizers chapter, let each bite be a celebration—an affirmation that snacking can be both delicious and healthful. These recipes not only cater to your cravings but also ensure that every snack is a note in the symphony of well-being, allowing women to savor each moment of indulgence with a mindful and health-conscious twist.

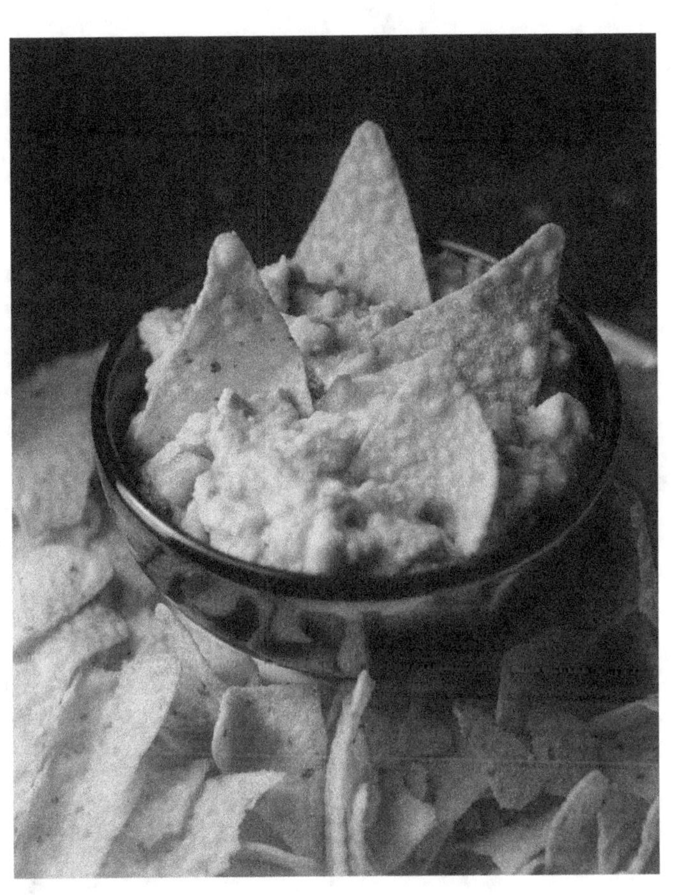

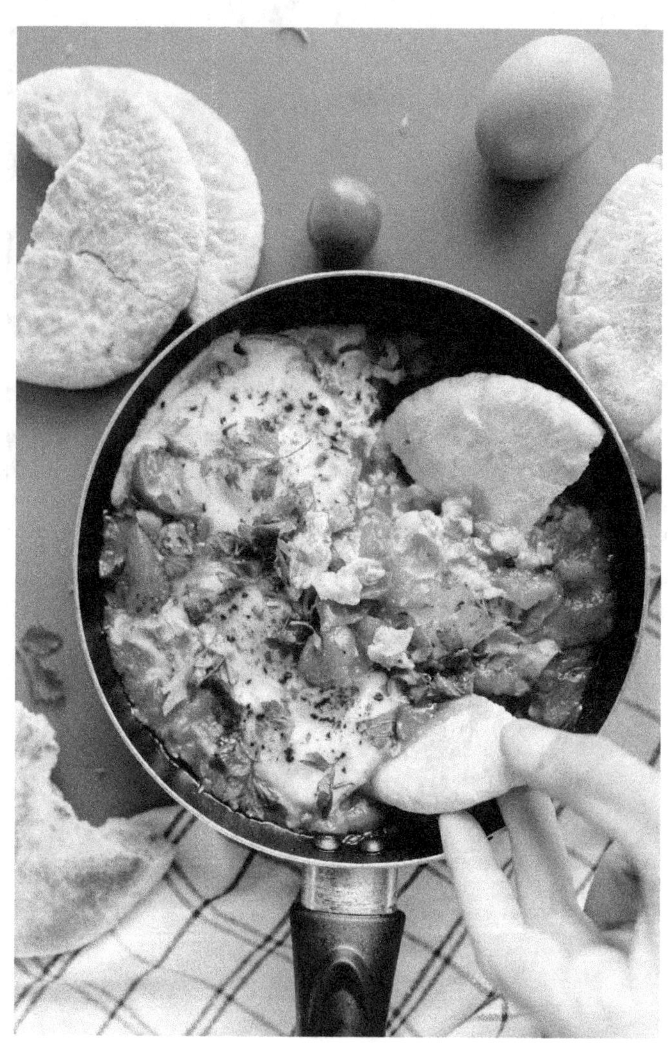

CHAPTER SIX

Sweets & Treats: A Symphony of Guilt-Free Indulgence for Women

In the orchestration of a woman's day, Sweets & Treats emerge as the sweet crescendo—a moment to indulge without compromise, to savor the joy of decadence while nurturing the body with healthful ingredients. "Harmony on the Plate: A Plant-Based Cookbook for Women" weaves a captivating chapter on Sweets & Treats, where each recipe is a delightful note in the symphony of healthful indulgence, tailored to empower and satiate women's cravings.

1. Decadent Desserts without Compromise: Nourishing the Sweet Tooth

Step into a world where sweetness knows no guilt with Decadent Desserts without Compromise. The Chocolate Avocado Mousse is a velvety delight that marries the rich creaminess of avocados with the deep flavors of cocoa, creating a luxurious treat that satisfies the sweet tooth while embracing healthful fats. For a fruity escape, the Berry Parfait layers vibrant berries with coconut yogurt and a sprinkle of granola, offering a refreshing yet indulgent dessert experience. These decadent desserts redefine the notion of sweet indulgence, proving that healthful choices can be synonymous with divine flavors.

2. Fruit-Infused Indulgences: Nature's Bounty in Every Bite

Sweets & Treats become a celebration of nature's bounty with Fruit-Infused Indulgences that showcase the natural sweetness of fresh fruits. The Mango Coconut Chia Pudding introduces layers of ripe mango, coconut-infused chia pudding, and a drizzle of honey—a tropical symphony in a jar. For a refreshing twist, the Watermelon Mint Sorbet offers a cool and revitalizing treat that combines the hydrating properties of watermelon with the invigorating essence of mint. These fruit-infused indulgences not only satisfy sugar cravings but also provide a plethora of vitamins and antioxidants, making dessert a guilt-free celebration of nature's sweetness.

3. Healthy Baking Simplified: Wholesome Goodness without Complication

Baking takes on a healthful and simplified persona in "Harmony on the Plate," offering a collection of treats that embody Wholesome Goodness without Complication. The Almond Flour Banana Bread combines the nutty richness of almond flour with the sweetness of ripe bananas, creating a moist and satisfying treat. For a nutty crunch, the Oatmeal Walnut Cookies showcase the heartiness of oats and the richness of walnuts, offering a wholesome alternative to traditional cookies. These baked delights redefine the art of baking, proving that healthful treats can be both simple and deeply satisfying.

4. Blissful Smoothie Popsicles: A Cool and Nourishing Delight

Satisfy your sweet cravings with a refreshing twist through Blissful Smoothie Popsicles. The Blueberry Mint Yogurt Pops blend the antioxidant power of blueberries with the cooling essence of mint, creating a delightful frozen treat that soothes and indulges. For a tropical escape, the Pineapple Coconut Chia Pops infuse the creaminess of coconut with the tropical sweetness of pineapple, offering a guilt-free popsicle experience. These cool delights not only provide relief on a warm day but also bring healthful ingredients to the forefront, making them a guilt-free option for women seeking a sweet and refreshing treat.

5. Healthy Nut Butter Cups: Nutty Richness, Minus the Guilt

Indulge in the nutty richness of Healthy Nut Butter Cups, a guilt-free alternative to satisfy your chocolate cravings. The Almond Butter Chocolate Cups combine the velvety richness of dark chocolate with the creaminess of almond butter, creating a bite-sized treat that delights the senses. For a crunchy twist, the Peanut Butter Crunch Cups introduce a layer of wholesome granola, adding texture to the smoothness of peanut butter and chocolate. These nut butter cups not only cater to your sweet tooth but also provide a source of plant-based proteins and healthy fats, offering a delightful balance of flavor and nutrition.

As you explore the recipes in the Sweets & Treats chapter, let each bite be a celebration—an affirmation that indulgence can coexist with healthful living. These recipes not only satisfy cravings but also prove that every sweet moment can be a harmonious blend of decadence and nourishment, allowing women to enjoy the symphony of flavors that come with guilt-free indulgence.

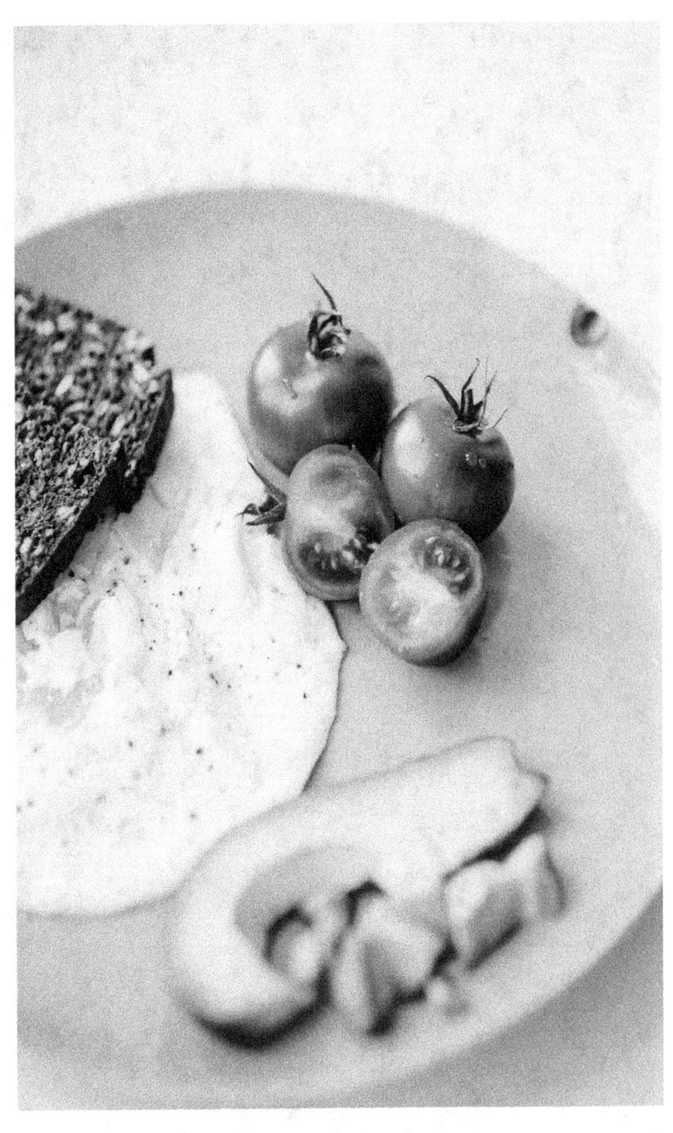

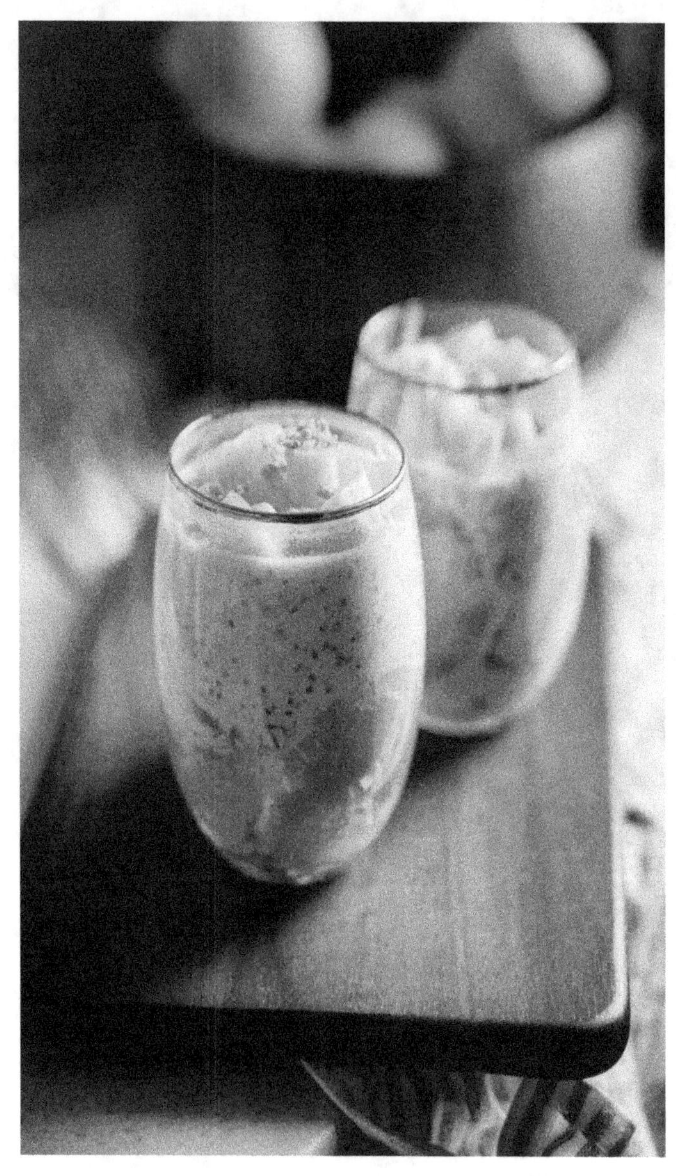

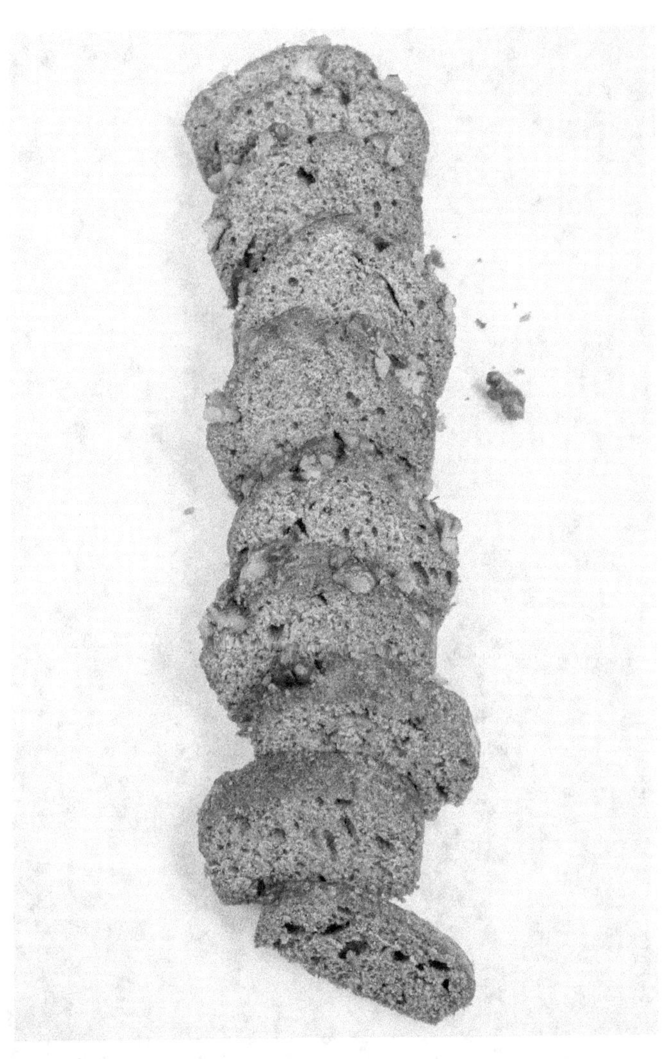

49

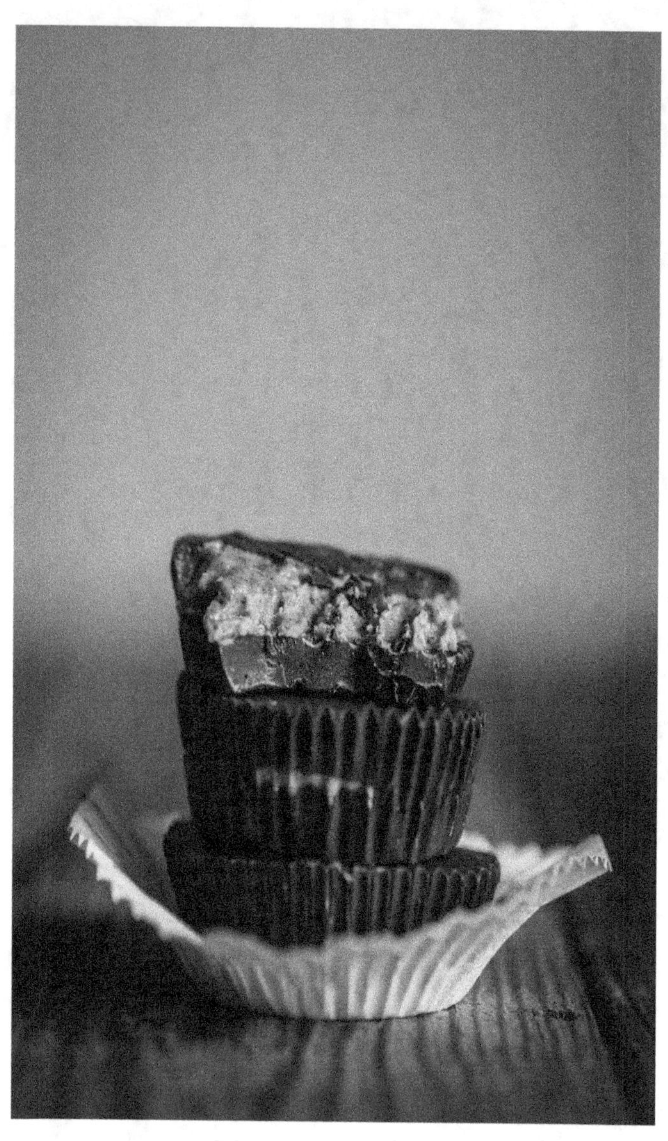

CHAPTER SEVEN

Beverages & Smoothies: A Symphony of Refreshment for Women's Well-being

In the daily melody of a woman's life, Beverages & Smoothies emerge as the refreshing interlude—a moment to hydrate, revitalize, and infuse the body with healthful goodness. "Harmony on the Plate: A Plant-Based Cookbook for Women" orchestrates a captivating chapter on Beverages & Smoothies, where each recipe is a flavorful note in the symphony of well-being, tailored to empower and nourish women.

1. Revitalizing Morning Elixirs: A Harmonious Start to the Day

Kickstart your day with Revitalizing Morning Elixirs, where each sip becomes a celebration of healthful hydration. The Green Goddess Detox Smoothie combines leafy greens, cucumber, and refreshing mint for a nutrient-packed elixir that invigorates and cleanses. For a tropical twist, the Pineapple Ginger Turmeric Smoothie infuses the anti-inflammatory benefits of turmeric with the tropical sweetness of pineapple and a hint of zing from ginger. These morning elixirs not only awaken your senses but also provide a burst of vitamins and antioxidants to fuel the day ahead.

2. Hydrating Infusions: Nature's Quench for Thirsty Souls

Quench your thirst with Hydrating Infusions that transform water into a symphony of flavors. The Cucumber Mint Infused Water embraces the cooling essence of cucumber and the invigorating aroma of mint, turning hydration into a refreshing experience. For a burst of citrusy delight, the Lemon Raspberry Basil Infused Water combines the zing of lemon with the sweetness of raspberries and the herbal notes of basil. These hydrating infusions not only promote water intake but also elevate your hydration experience with the flavors of nature.

3. Nourishing Smoothie Bowls: A Feast for the Senses and Body

Bask in the decadence of Nourishing Smoothie Bowls, where each spoonful is a journey into the heart of healthful living. The Acai Berry Bliss Bowl combines the antioxidant-rich acai berry with an assortment of vibrant fruits and a sprinkle of granola for a visual and culinary masterpiece. For a protein-packed option, the Protein-Packed Green Smoothie Bowl introduces plant-based protein sources like spinach, almond butter, and chia seeds. These smoothie bowls are not just a feast for the senses but also a powerhouse of nutrients that leave you feeling satisfied and energized.

4. Invigorating Iced Teas: Cool Sips with a Burst of Flavor

Cool down with Invigorating Iced Teas that blend the comforting ritual of tea with the revitalizing essence of chilled refreshment. The Berry Hibiscus Iced Tea infuses the floral notes of hibiscus with the sweetness of mixed berries, creating a vibrant and antioxidant-rich beverage. For a tropical escape, the Pineapple Mint Green Iced Tea marries the crispness of green tea with the tropical sweetness of pineapple and the cooling touch of mint. These iced teas not only quench your thirst but also provide a refreshing and healthful alternative to sugary beverages.

5. Post-Workout Protein Shakes: Fueling Recovery with Plant Power

After a workout, replenish your energy with Post-Workout Protein Shakes that harness the power of plant-based proteins. The Berry Blast Protein Shake blends berries with plant-based protein powder, almond milk, and a touch of nut butter for a delicious and protein-packed recovery drink. For a green twist, the Kale and Pineapple Protein Smoothie combines the leafy goodness of kale with the tropical sweetness of pineapple, creating a refreshing and nutrient-dense shake. These protein shakes not only aid in muscle recovery but also offer a delicious and healthful way to refuel after exercise.

As you explore the recipes in the Beverages & Smoothies chapter, let each sip be a celebration—an affirmation that hydration and refreshment can be a flavorful journey. These recipes not only offer a symphony of flavors but also showcase the versatility and vibrancy that plant-based ingredients bring to your cup. In every beverage and smoothie, discover the harmonious blend of well-being and indulgence, allowing women to sip their way to vitality and healthful enjoyment.

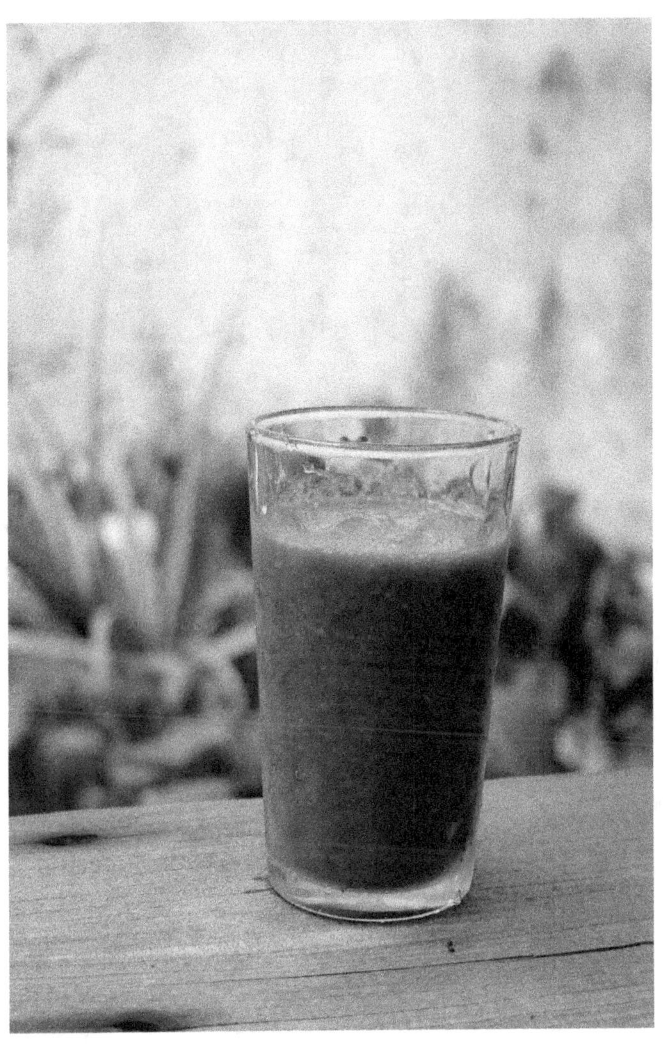

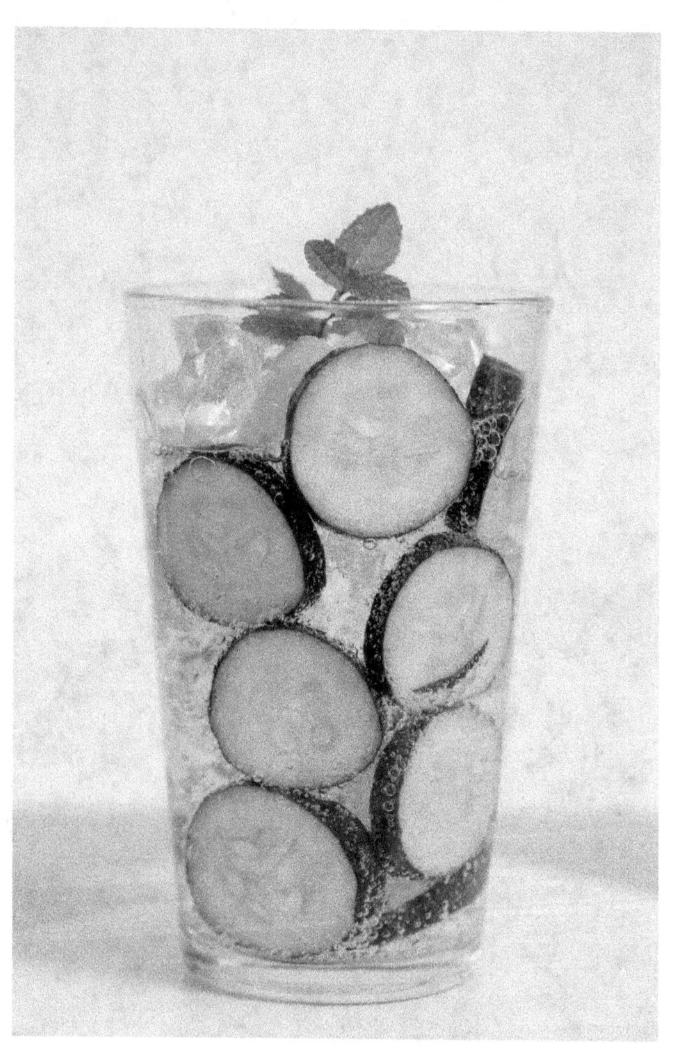

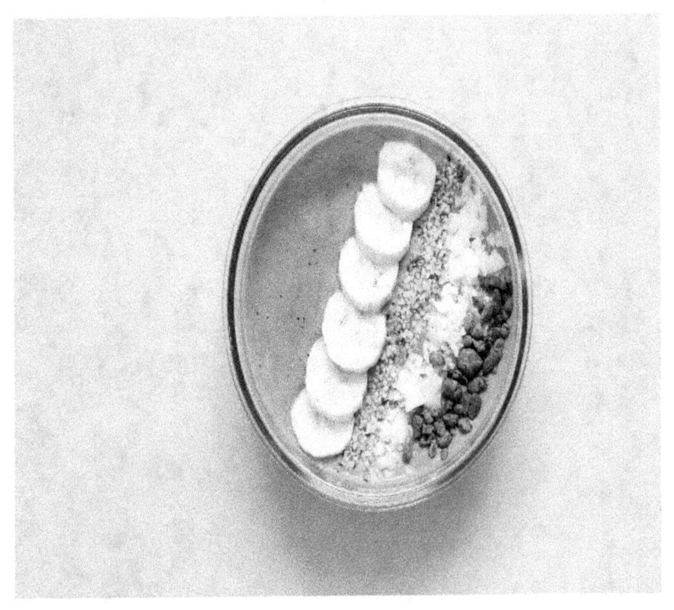

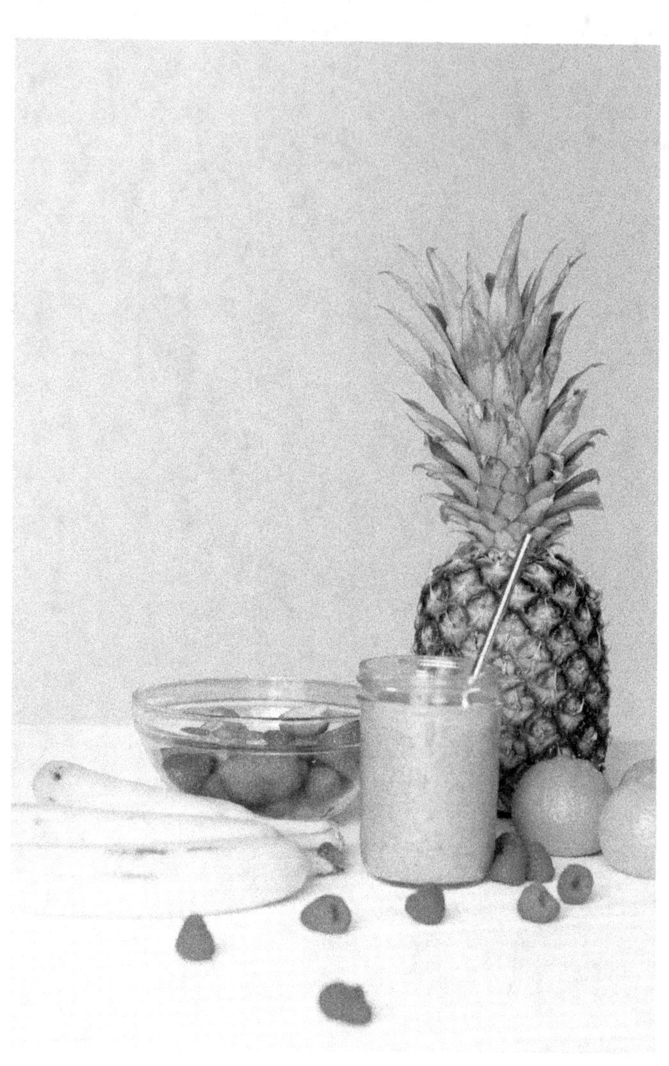

CHAPTER EIGHT

Meal Planning Made Easy: A Week of Wholesome Delights

Welcome to the heart of simplicity and nourishment – "Meal Planning Made Easy" in "Harmony on the Plate: A Plant-Based Cookbook for Women." This comprehensive guide not only unveils the secrets of crafting weekly plant-based meal plans but also shares invaluable tips for efficient batch cooking. Let's embark on a culinary journey where every meal is a symphony of flavors, health, and ease.

Creating Weekly Plant-Based Meal Plans: A Symphony of Variety

Unlock the art of creating Weekly Plant-Based Meal Plans, transforming your week into a culinary adventure filled with diverse and healthful delights. Each day becomes a unique note, contributing to the harmonious composition of nourishment. "Harmony on the Plate" offers an array of delectable plant-based recipes tailored to suit every palate, from vibrant salads to hearty stews, ensuring each day is a celebration of health and flavor.

Monday: Meatless Marvels

Start the week with the freshness of a Mediterranean Chickpea Salad.
Dive into the robust flavors of a Spicy Lentil and Vegetable Stew for dinner.

Tuesday: Taco Night Fiesta

Embrace the fiesta with Black Bean and Veggie Tacos.
Conclude the night with a refreshing Mango Avocado Salsa.

Wednesday: Wholesome Grain Bowls

Savor the goodness of a Quinoa and Roasted Vegetable Bowl.
Elevate your evening with a protein-packed Teriyaki Tofu Grain Bowl.

Thursday: Pasta Paradise

Delight in a Creamy Tomato Basil Pasta for a comforting lunch.
Indulge in a Pesto Zucchini Noodles dish for a light and flavorful dinner.

Friday: Fusion Flavors

Enjoy a Chickpea and Vegetable Stir-Fry for a burst of Asian-inspired flavors.
Conclude the week with a hearty Sweet Potato and Black Bean Burrito Bowl.

Tips for Efficient Batch Cooking: A Culinary Symphony in Advance

Efficiency takes center stage with Tips for Efficient Batch Cooking, a strategy that transforms your kitchen into a harmonious space of preparedness and simplicity. Dive into the art of preparing larger quantities of key components to streamline your daily cooking endeavors. These tips ensure a bounty of delicious meals without the stress of daily preparations.

Prep Your Ingredients in Batches:

Chop vegetables, marinate proteins, and measure spices in advance for quick and efficient cooking during the week.

Cook Grains and Legumes in Bulk:

Prepare a large batch of quinoa, brown rice, or lentils to use as versatile base ingredients throughout the week.

Roast a Medley of Vegetables:

Roast a variety of vegetables, such as sweet potatoes, bell peppers, and zucchini, for quick additions to salads, bowls, or wraps.

Make Flavorful Sauces and Dressings:

Whip up flavorful sauces and dressings that can be stored and used to enhance the taste of your dishes during the week.

Portion and Freeze:

Portion meals into individual containers and freeze for grab-and-go convenience, ensuring you have healthful options readily available.

Harmony on the Plate: Where Efficiency Meets Flavor

"Harmony on the Plate" redefines meal planning as a seamless blend of variety, health, and ease. With Weekly Plant-Based Meal Plans and Tips for Efficient Batch Cooking, every woman can embark on a culinary journey that transcends the ordinary. As you savor the symphony of flavors in each thoughtfully planned meal, let it be a reminder that nourishment can be both delicious and effortlessly attainable. Embrace the ease, relish the variety, and discover the joy that comes with a well-crafted and efficient approach to meal planning in the heart of "Harmony on the Plate."

CHAPTER NINE

Special Occasions: A Symphony of Celebration with Elegant Plant-Based Menus

Step into the world of refined celebration with "Harmony on the Plate: A Plant-Based Cookbook for Women," where special occasions unfold as a symphony of exquisite flavors, elegant presentations, and plant-based indulgence. This chapter unveils Elegant Plant-Based Menus crafted to elevate celebrations and holiday feasts, infusing every moment with the joy of healthful and delightful dining.

Elegant Plant-Based Menus: Crafting Culinary Masterpieces

Experience the art of culinary mastery with Elegant Plant-Based Menus designed for those extraordinary moments. Each menu is a meticulously curated composition of flavors, textures, and visual delights, transforming celebrations into unforgettable experiences.

- **Menu 1: Symphony of Spring Soiree**
    - Appetizer: Asparagus and Cashew Cream Tartlets
    - Main Course: Lemon Risotto with Pea Shoots and Mint
    - Dessert: Strawberry Basil Sorbet with Balsamic Reduction

- **Menu 2: Mediterranean Feast Under the Stars**
    - Appetizer: Roasted Red Pepper and Walnut Dip with Pita Chips
    - Main Course: Stuffed Grape Leaves with Lemon-Dill Tofu
    - Dessert: Olive Oil and Orange Blossom Cake
- **Menu 3: Winter Wonderland Gala**
    - Appetizer: Butternut Squash and Sage Crostini
    - Main Course: Wild Mushroom and Truffle Risotto
    - Dessert: Spiced Poached Pears with Pomegranate Reduction

Holiday Feasts with a Plant-Based Twist: A Joyful Culinary Journey

Celebrate the holiday season with a plant-based twist, where familiar traditions meet innovative and healthful ingredients. The Holiday Feasts featured in "Harmony on the Plate" reimagine festive dining with decadence and a plant-powered touch.

- **Feast 1: Thanksgiving Harvest Extravaganza**
    - Appetizer: Pumpkin and Sage Cashew Cheese Crostini
    - Main Course: Lentil and Mushroom Stuffed Acorn Squash
    - Dessert: Maple Pecan Pie with Coconut Whipped Cream

- **Feast 2: Christmas Elegance with a Twist**
    - Appetizer: Cranberry and Walnut Stuffed Mushrooms
    - Main Course: Herb-Crusted Tofurkey with Rosemary Gravy
    - Dessert: Chocolate Peppermint Mousse Cake
- **Feast 3: New Year's Eve Sparkling Soirée**
    - Appetizer: Avocado and Mango Tartare with Wonton Crisps
    - Main Course: Champagne Risotto with Truffle Oil
    - Dessert: Raspberry Champagne Sorbet with Edible Gold Flakes

Culinary Artistry: A Feast for the Senses

Experience culinary artistry as each menu unfolds, presenting a feast for the senses. From the first bite of an appetizer to the last spoonful of dessert, these Elegant Plant-Based Menus redefine celebration, proving that healthful dining can be synonymous with gourmet indulgence.

A Plant-Based Celebration: Where Joy Meets Wellness

In "Harmony on the Plate," special occasions transcend the ordinary, becoming a celebration where joy meets wellness. Elegant Plant-Based Menus and Holiday Feasts with a Plant-Based Twist guide you through an extraordinary journey of refined flavors, thoughtful presentations, and healthful delight. Whether you're hosting a spring soiree, a winter gala, or a holiday feast, let each menu be a reminder that plant-based dining is not just a choice—it's an elevated and joyous celebration of life, love, and the art of savoring every exquisite moment.

CHAPTER TEN

Essential Tips for Women's Well-Being: Nourishing the Body and Mind

In the pursuit of holistic well-being, women play a central role in nurturing their bodies and minds. "Harmony on the Plate: A Plant-Based Cookbook for Women" unveils a comprehensive guide featuring Essential Tips for Women's Well-Being. From thoughtful nutritional considerations to seamlessly incorporating plant-based choices into daily life, these tips empower women to embrace a lifestyle that harmonizes with their health, vitality, and overall happiness.

Nutritional Considerations: Fueling the Female Body with Purpose

Balanced Macronutrients:
Ensure a balanced intake of macronutrients—proteins, carbohydrates, and fats. For optimal health, women should include lean plant-based proteins, whole grains, and healthy fats such as avocados, nuts, and seeds in their daily diet. This balance supports energy levels, muscle health, and hormonal balance.

Calcium and Vitamin D:
Prioritize sources of calcium and vitamin D for bone health. Plant-based options like fortified plant milks,

tofu, leafy greens, and exposure to sunlight contribute to maintaining strong and healthy bones, a crucial consideration for women's well-being.

Iron-Rich Foods:

Pay attention to iron-rich foods to support energy levels and prevent iron deficiency. Plant-based sources such as lentils, beans, spinach, and fortified cereals offer a readily absorbable form of iron, ensuring women meet their nutritional needs.

Omega-3 Fatty Acids:

Incorporate omega-3 fatty acids, vital for heart and brain health. Chia seeds, flaxseeds, walnuts, and algae-based supplements provide plant-based sources of these essential fats, contributing to overall well-being.

Fiber-Rich Choices:

Prioritize fiber-rich foods to support digestion and overall gut health. Whole grains, legumes, fruits, and vegetables offer a plethora of fiber, promoting satiety and supporting a healthy digestive system.

Hydration:

Stay well-hydrated to support bodily functions, skin health, and overall vitality. Water, herbal teas, and infused water with fruits and herbs provide refreshing and hydrating options for women seeking optimal well-being.

Incorporating Plant-Based Choices into Daily Life: A Lifestyle of Harmony

Gradual Transitions:

Embrace plant-based choices gradually, allowing for a smooth transition. Start by incorporating more fruits, vegetables, and plant-based proteins into meals, exploring diverse flavors and textures.

Colorful Plate Philosophy:

Adhere to the "Colorful Plate" philosophy, ensuring a diverse array of fruits and vegetables in every meal. The vibrant hues represent a spectrum of nutrients, supporting immune function, skin health, and overall vitality.

Meal Planning with Purpose:

Engage in mindful meal planning, creating balanced and satisfying plant-based meals. Plan a variety of dishes that include different textures, flavors, and nutrient profiles, enhancing the overall dining experience.

Exploration of Plant-Based Proteins:

Explore a variety of plant-based protein sources to ensure nutritional adequacy. Incorporate legumes, tofu, tempeh, seitan, and plant-based protein powders into meals to meet protein requirements for muscle health and overall well-being

Plant-Powered Snacking:

Opt for plant-powered snacks that provide sustained energy and nourishment between meals. Fresh fruit, nuts, seeds, and veggie sticks with hummus or nut butter make for satisfying and healthful snack choices.

Mindful Dining Habits:

Cultivate mindful dining habits, paying attention to hunger and fullness cues. This practice supports a healthy relationship with food, preventing overeating and promoting mindful enjoyment of each meal.

Educational Resources:

Seek educational resources and recipes that align with a plant-based lifestyle. Empower yourself with knowledge about plant-based nutrition, discovering new recipes and culinary techniques that make the transition enjoyable and sustainable.

Conclusion: A Symphony of Well-Being

In the tapestry of women's well-being, the Essential Tips presented in "Harmony on the Plate" offer a symphony of guidance for both nourishing the body and incorporating plant-based choices into daily life. By considering key nutritional aspects and seamlessly integrating plant-based options, women can embark on a journey towards vibrant health, sustainable vitality, and a harmonious balance between nourishment and joy. With each thoughtful choice, women can contribute to their well-being, creating a lifestyle that resonates with the beautiful harmony of a life well-lived.

Conclusion: The Journey Continues - Sustaining a Plant-Based Lifestyle

As we draw the final notes of "Harmony on the Plate: A Plant-Based Cookbook for Women," it's not just the end of a book; it's the beginning of a transformative journey—a journey towards sustained well-being, mindful choices, and a harmonious relationship with the nourishment our bodies deserve. The pages may end, but the symphony of a plant-based lifestyle resonates beyond the cookbook, echoing in every healthful choice, in every delicious plant-based creation, and in the vibrant well-being that awaits.

Embrace the Symphony of Choices:

As you navigate the path of a plant-based lifestyle, remember that every choice is a note in your unique symphony. Embrace the vibrancy of colorful plant-based plates, savor the richness of nutrient-dense foods, and relish the diverse flavors that nature generously provides. Your journey is a celebration, and each meal is an opportunity to compose a masterpiece of health and joy.

Sustainability Beyond the Plate:

The sustainability of a plant-based lifestyle extends beyond the plate. Consider the environmental impact of your choices—reduce, reuse, and recycle. Support local farmers and markets, choose sustainably sourced ingredients, and let your commitment to well-being ripple into a positive influence for the planet.

Cultivate Mindful Eating:

In the hustle of daily life, pause to cultivate mindful eating. Turn meals into moments of presence, appreciating the textures, aromas, and flavors. Mindful eating not only enhances digestion but also deepens your connection with the nourishment your body receives, fostering a sense of gratitude and well-being.

Explore and Innovate:

Let curiosity be your compass. Explore the vast landscape of plant-based ingredients, discover new recipes, and innovate in the kitchen. The world of plant-based cooking is an ever-expanding canvas, and your culinary journey is an opportunity for continuous exploration, creativity, and delightful surprises.

Celebrate Progress, Not Perfection:

In your pursuit of a plant-based lifestyle, celebrate progress rather than perfection. Recognize that every step you take towards mindful and healthful choices is a victory. Embrace the flexibility of your journey, acknowledging that small, sustainable changes lead to lasting well-being.

Connect with a Community:

Build connections with like-minded individuals who share your passion for plant-based living. Join online communities, attend local events, and exchange experiences. A supportive community becomes a source of inspiration, guidance, and shared joy in the journey towards health and vitality.

Listen to Your Body's Symphony:

Your body has its own symphony—a unique composition of needs, preferences, and signals. Listen attentively. Pay heed to hunger and fullness cues, observe how your body responds to different foods, and tailor your plant-based choices to create a harmonious melody that resonates with your individual well-being.

Gratitude for Every Bite:

As you savor each bite of a well-prepared plant-based meal, let gratitude accompany your dining experience. Acknowledge the effort put into cultivating, preparing, and presenting the nourishing ingredients on your plate. A heart filled with gratitude transforms the act of eating into a soul-nourishing ritual.

The Journey Continues:

In conclusion, "Harmony on the Plate" is not a destination but a guide—an invitation to a lifestyle where health, joy, and plant-based choices dance in unison. The journey continues with each choice you make, each meal you prepare, and each moment you dedicate to the well-being of your body and the planet.

As you embark on the ongoing symphony of a plant-based lifestyle, let the wisdom gleaned from these pages resonate in your daily life. May your journey be filled with vibrant health, culinary delights, and a deep connection to the harmony that comes from choosing well, living well, and nurturing both body and soul. The final refrain of this book is not an end—it's an invitation to continue composing the beautiful melody of a plant-based life. The journey continues, and the stage is set for a lifetime of well-being, joy, and the harmonious dance of plant-based living.

DAILY REMARK

Day	Recipes	Remark

		76

www.ingramcontent.com/pod-product-compliance
Lightning Source LLC
Chambersburg PA
CBHW061013260726

48661CB00005B/2179